Invasive Plants Guide for Beginners

Combating Invasive Plants

By

Declan Eystein
Copyright@2023

Table of Contents

CHAPTER 1

Introduction

1.1 What Are Invasive Plants

Invasive plants, often referred to as invasive species or weeds, are non-native plants that have been introduced to a new environment, where they aggressively spread and disrupt the balance of native ecosystems. These plants are considered invasive because they possess certain characteristics that enable them to outcompete native vegetation, reproduce rapidly, and thrive in their new surroundings. Invasive plants can cause significant ecological, economic, and even health-related problems, making them a matter of critical concern for environmentalists, scientists, land managers, and conservationists worldwide.

Key characteristics of invasive plants include:

1. **Rapid Growth:** Invasive plants often grow faster than native species, allowing them to quickly establish themselves in an area.

2. **High Reproductive Rates:** They produce a large number of seeds, fruits, or vegetative propagules, enhancing their ability to colonize new habitats.

3. **Lack of Natural Predators:** In their non-native environments, invasive plants are often free from the natural predators and diseases that would typically

keep their populations in check in their native range.

4. **Adaptability:** Invasive plants are highly adaptable to a variety of environmental conditions, making them resilient and capable of thriving in diverse ecosystems.

5. **Alteration of Ecosystems:** They can alter soil chemistry, water availability, and other ecological factors, negatively impacting native plants, wildlife, and ecosystem functions.

Examples of invasive plants vary by region but may include species like Japanese Knotweed, European Buckthorn, Purple Loosestrife, and many others. These plants, once established, can dominate landscapes, displace native flora, and disrupt the delicate relationships that exist within ecosystems.

1.2 Why Should Beginners Learn About Invasive Plants

Learning about invasive plants is essential for beginners and, indeed, for everyone, because of the far-reaching implications of invasive species on our environment, economy, and even human health. Here are several compelling reasons why beginners should make it a priority to understand and engage with invasive plant issues:

1. Environmental Conservation: Invasive plants pose a severe threat to natural ecosystems. By learning about them, beginners can actively participate in efforts to protect and restore native habitats. Understanding the impact of invasive species is crucial for preserving biodiversity and maintaining the health of our natural environment.

2. Economic Impact: Invasive plants can have substantial economic consequences. They can damage agricultural crops, increase the cost of pest control, and reduce property values. Learning to identify and address invasive plants can help communities save money and resources.

3. Personal and Public Health: Some invasive plants are not only detrimental to the environment but also harmful to human health. For instance, certain invasive plants can cause allergies, skin irritation, or even poisonings. Knowledge about these plants can help individuals protect themselves and their communities.

4. Responsible Land Stewardship: For landowners and gardeners, understanding invasive plants is essential for responsible land management. It enables them to make informed choices about landscaping, gardening, and restoration efforts, promoting the use of native plants and sustainable practices.

5. Community Involvement: Learning about invasive plants provides an opportunity for beginners to engage with their communities. Many regions have volunteer programs and citizen science initiatives focused on invasive species management. This involvement fosters a sense of environmental responsibility and community connection.

6. Future Impact: As the effects of climate change become more pronounced, invasive species may become an even greater challenge. Beginners who educate themselves about invasive plants today will be better equipped to address future ecological changes and mitigate their impacts.

Invasive plants are not merely an academic pursuit; it is a crucial aspect of responsible environmental stewardship. Beginners who take the time to learn about invasive plants are taking a proactive step toward preserving the natural world, protecting local economies, and ensuring the well-being of future generations. It empowers individuals to be informed and engaged citizens in the ongoing battle against invasive species, ultimately contributing to the sustainability of our planet.

CHAPTER 2

Understanding Invasive Plants

2.1 Definition and Characteristics

Definition: Invasive plants, also known as invasive species or weeds, are non-native plant species that, when introduced to a new environment, exhibit aggressive growth and spread patterns, often outcompeting native vegetation and disrupting the balance of ecosystems.

2.2 Common Misconceptions

There are several misconceptions about invasive plants that can hinder effective management and understanding. Addressing these misconceptions is crucial:

Misconception 1: All Non-Native Plants Are Invasive: Not all non-native plants are invasive. While many non-native plants can coexist harmlessly with native species, invasive plants possess specific characteristics that enable them to become invasive and problematic.

Misconception 2: Invasive Plants Are Always Easy to Spot: Invasive plants don't always look out of place. Some can resemble native species closely, making identification challenging. It's essential to learn the distinguishing features of both native and invasive species.

Misconception 3: Invasive Plants Are Only a Problem in Natural Areas: Invasive plants can thrive in a variety of environments, including urban and suburban areas. They can impact gardens, parks, and agricultural lands as well as natural ecosystems.

Misconception 4: Removing Invasive Plants Solves the Problem: Eradicating invasive plants can be challenging and may require ongoing management. The focus should also be on restoring native habitats to prevent reinvasion.

Misconception 5: Invasive Plants Are Always Bad: While invasive plants are generally detrimental to ecosystems, some may have beneficial uses, such as for erosion control or medicinal purposes. However, these cases are exceptions, and the overall impact is negative.

2.3 Impact on Ecosystems

Invasive plants have profound and often detrimental impacts on ecosystems:

1. **Displacement of Native Species:** Invasive plants can outcompete native vegetation for resources like sunlight, water, and nutrients, leading to a decline in native plant populations.

2. **Altered Habitat Structure:** They can change the physical structure of habitats, making

them less suitable for native wildlife, including birds, insects, and other animals that depend on specific vegetation.

3. **Disruption of Ecological Relationships:** Invasive plants can disrupt the ecological relationships between native plants and their pollinators, herbivores, and seed dispersers, affecting the entire food web.

4. **Loss of Biodiversity:** As invasive plants proliferate, they reduce plant diversity and, consequently, the diversity of animals and microorganisms that depend on native plants.

5. **Increased Fire Risk:** Some invasive plants, like cheatgrass, are highly flammable and can

increase the risk of wildfires in certain ecosystems.

6. **Altered Soil Chemistry:** Invasive plants can change soil chemistry by affecting nutrient cycling, which can have cascading effects on other plant species.

7. **Economic Costs:** The impact of invasive plants extends beyond ecosystems. They can harm agriculture, forestry, and tourism industries, leading to significant economic losses.

Understanding the definition, characteristics, misconceptions, and ecological impact of invasive plants is vital for effective conservation and management efforts. Awareness and education are key tools in mitigating the negative effects of invasive

species and preserving native
ecosystems.

CHAPTER 3

Identifying Invasive Plants

3.1 Some benefits of Invasive Plants

While invasive plants are generally considered harmful and detrimental to ecosystems, it's essential to acknowledge that some individuals might perceive certain benefits associated with them. However, these benefits are often outweighed by the negative impacts. Here are a few potential benefits of invasive plants, along with important caveats:

1. **Erosion Control:** Some invasive plants, such as kudzu,

can form dense ground cover that may help reduce soil erosion in certain situations. However, their aggressive growth can also lead to other ecological problems.

2. **Medicinal and Cultural Uses:** A few invasive plants have traditional or medicinal uses in certain cultures. For instance, some invasive plants like garlic mustard have culinary or herbal applications. However, these uses do not justify their invasive behavior or ecological harm.

3. **Wildlife Habitat:** Invasive plants may provide temporary food sources or shelter for wildlife. However, these benefits are often short-lived, and the long-term consequences

of invasive species outweigh any advantages.

4. **Aesthetic Appeal:** Invasive plants might have attractive flowers or foliage that some individuals find appealing in landscaping. Still, their potential to escape cultivation and invade natural areas raises significant ecological concerns.

5. **Low Maintenance:** Invasive plants can be hardy and require minimal maintenance in gardens or landscaping. However, this convenience can come at the cost of local ecosystems.

It's important to approach these perceived benefits with caution and awareness of the broader ecological context. The negative ecological impacts of invasive plants, including habitat destruction, displacement of native species, and disruption of ecosystems, far outweigh any potential advantages. Understanding the full picture of invasive plant effects is essential for informed decision-making and responsible land management.

CHAPTER 4

The Most Notorious Invasive Plants

4.1 Japanese Knotweed

Japanese Knotweed (Reynoutria japonica) is one of the most notorious and invasive plant species in many regions, particularly in North America and Europe. Here are some key characteristics and impacts of Japanese Knotweed:

- **Identification:** Japanese Knotweed is a perennial herbaceous plant with bamboo-like stems that can reach heights of 10 feet (3 meters). It has distinct, heart-shaped leaves and clusters of small, white to pale green flowers.

- **Invasive Behavior:** Japanese Knotweed forms dense thickets that outcompete native vegetation, reducing biodiversity. Its aggressive root system can damage infrastructure, such as buildings and roads.

- **Spread:** The plant reproduces through rhizomes and can regenerate from small root fragments. This makes it extremely challenging to control.

- **Impact on Ecosystems:** Japanese Knotweed alters soil chemistry and can lead to soil erosion. It also disrupts aquatic ecosystems when it invades riverbanks and wetlands.

- **Management:** Effective management typically involves a combination of mechanical removal, herbicide treatment, and ongoing monitoring due to its persistence.

4.2 Kudzu

Kudzu (Pueraria montana var. lobata) is often referred to as "The Vine That Ate the South" due to its rapid and extensive spread in the southeastern United States. Here are some key features and impacts of Kudzu:

- **Identification:** Kudzu is a high-climbing, perennial vine with large, three-lobed leaves and clusters of purple flowers. It can cover and smother entire trees, buildings, and structures.

- **Invasive Behavior:** Kudzu is known for its incredibly fast growth, with vines that can grow up to one foot (30 centimeters) per day. It shades out native plants, leading to reduced biodiversity.

- **Spread:** Kudzu reproduces both through seeds and vegetative propagation. It spreads rapidly along roadsides, forests, and disturbed areas.

- **Impact on Ecosystems:** Kudzu alters natural landscapes, disrupts forest canopies, and may increase the risk of wildfires due to its flammability.

- **Management:** Managing Kudzu requires a combination of mechanical removal, herbicide treatments, and long-term monitoring efforts.

4.3 Purple Loosestrife

Purple Loosestrife (Lythrum salicaria) is another highly invasive plant, primarily affecting wetlands and riparian areas. Here are some key features and impacts of Purple Loosestrife:

- **Identification:** Purple Loosestrife is a perennial herb with tall spikes of purple-pink flowers and lance-shaped leaves. Its distinctive flowers make it easy to identify.

- **Invasive Behavior:** This plant forms dense stands that outcompete native wetland vegetation, reducing habitat quality for wildlife.

- **Spread:** Purple Loosestrife reproduces prolifically through both seeds and vegetative means, allowing it to colonize wetland areas rapidly.

- **Impact on Ecosystems:** It can transform wetland ecosystems by displacing native plants, reducing plant diversity, and negatively affecting wetland-dependent wildlife.

- **Management:** Management strategies include biological control through the introduction of natural enemies (biocontrol agents), herbicide application, and manual removal.

4.4 Common Buckthorn

Common Buckthorn (Rhamnus cathartica) is a highly invasive shrub or small tree that has become a significant problem in various regions. Here are some key features and impacts of Common Buckthorn:

- **Identification:** Common Buckthorn typically grows to 10-25 feet (3-8 meters) in height. It has dark green, elliptical leaves and clusters of small, greenish-yellow flowers. The berries produced by this plant are glossy black when ripe.

- **Invasive Behavior:** Common Buckthorn forms dense thickets in forests, wetlands, and open areas. It leafs out earlier and retains its leaves later than many native plants, giving it a competitive advantage.

- **Spread:** It produces large quantities of berries, which are consumed by birds, allowing for widespread seed dispersal. Its ability to regenerate from the root system also contributes to its spread.

- **Impact on Ecosystems:** Common Buckthorn shades out native vegetation, disrupts forest understories, and reduces habitat quality for wildlife. It can alter soil chemistry and negatively impact soil microorganisms.

- **Management:** Management strategies include cutting and removing adult plants, especially before they produce berries, and the use of herbicides. Ongoing monitoring and control efforts are necessary due to its ability to resprout.

4.5 Mile-a-Minute Vine

Mile-a-Minute Vine (Persicaria perfoliata) is an extremely fast-growing, annual vine that can become a rampant invader in various ecosystems. Here are some key features and impacts of Mile-a-Minute Vine:

- **Identification:** Mile-a-Minute Vine is aptly named due to its rapid growth, with stems that can grow up to 6 inches (15 centimeters) per day. Its leaves are triangular and resemble those of the cucumber plant.

- **Invasive Behavior:** This vine forms dense mats that smother and shade out native vegetation, preventing the growth of other plants and reducing biodiversity.

- **Spread:** Mile-a-Minute Vine reproduces via seeds, which are spread by birds and other wildlife, as well as by its ability to root at nodes along the stem.

- **Impact on Ecosystems:** It can rapidly colonize disturbed areas, forests, and wetlands, disrupting the natural vegetation and ecological processes of these habitats.

- **Management:** Management strategies include mechanical removal, herbicide treatment, and preventing seed production by removing plants before they flower and produce seeds. Because of its rapid growth, frequent monitoring is necessary.

CHAPTER 5

How Invasive Plants Spread

5.1 Methods of Dispersal

Invasive plants employ various methods of dispersal to spread and establish themselves in new environments. Understanding these dispersal mechanisms is essential for managing and preventing their spread. Here are some common methods of dispersal used by invasive plants:

1. **Seeds:** Many invasive plants produce large quantities of seeds that can be dispersed by wind, water, animals, or human activity. Wind-dispersed seeds are often equipped with

structures like wings or parachutes to aid in their dispersal.

2. **Birds and Wildlife:** Birds and mammals play a significant role in seed dispersal. They eat the fruits of invasive plants and then spread the seeds through their droppings as they move about.

3. **Water:** Invasive plants in wetland areas often rely on water for seed dispersal. Seeds may float downstream in rivers or become lodged in the fur of animals that swim in water bodies.

4. **Human Activities:** Human activities are a primary vector for the spread of invasive plants. Seeds can attach to

clothing, footwear, vehicles, and equipment, allowing them to be transported to new locations inadvertently.

5. **Garden Plants:** Invasive plants are sometimes introduced into new areas intentionally as garden ornamentals. They can escape cultivation and establish self-sustaining populations in the wild.

6. **Vegetative Propagation:** Some invasive plants can reproduce vegetatively through fragments of roots, stems, or other plant parts. These fragments can be spread by activities like soil disturbance or mowing.

7. **Invasive Plants as Contaminants:** Invasive plants

can also be transported inadvertently as contaminants in agricultural products, soil, mulch, or other materials.

5.2 Preventing Spread in Your Area

Preventing the spread of invasive plants in your area is essential to protect native ecosystems and maintain biodiversity. Here are some steps you can take to help prevent the spread of invasive plants:

1. **Learn to Identify Invasive Plants:** Educate yourself about common invasive plants in your region. Knowing what to look for is the first step in prevention.

2. **Practice Good Garden Habits:** Be cautious when selecting and planting ornamental plants. Choose native or non-invasive species for your garden and landscaping projects.

3. **Clean Your Gear:** If you work or recreate in natural areas, make sure to clean your shoes, clothing, and equipment to remove seeds and plant fragments before leaving. This is particularly important for hikers, campers, and outdoor enthusiasts.

4. **Don't Move Firewood:** Avoid transporting firewood from one area to another, as it can carry invasive insects and plant pathogens.

5. **Support Local Regulations:**
   Be aware of and support local
   regulations and initiatives
   aimed at controlling invasive
   species. Participate in
   community clean-up efforts and
   invasive plant removal projects.

6. **Report Sightings:** If you spot
   invasive plants in your area,
   report them to local authorities
   or conservation organizations.
   Early detection and rapid
   response are key to preventing
   their establishment.

7. **Avoid Invasive Landscaping:**
   Be cautious when landscaping
   your property. Avoid planting
   invasive species, and remove
   any invasive plants that may
   already be present.

8. **Educate Others:** Share your knowledge about invasive plants with friends, family, and neighbors. Encourage responsible landscaping and land management practices in your community.

9. **Support Research and Conservation:** Consider supporting research and conservation efforts aimed at understanding and managing invasive species in your region.

Preventing the spread of invasive plants requires vigilance, education, and collective action. By taking steps to reduce the introduction and spread of invasive species, you can contribute to the preservation of native ecosystems and the protection of biodiversity.

CHAPTER 6

The Environmental Impact

6.1 Ecological Consequences

Invasive plants have far-reaching ecological consequences, often disrupting natural ecosystems in various ways:

- **Competition with Native Plants:** Invasive plants often outcompete native species for essential resources like sunlight, water, and nutrients.

This competition can lead to reduced biodiversity and alter the composition of plant communities.

- **Habitat Degradation:** As invasive plants spread and dominate ecosystems, they can transform habitats. They may alter soil chemistry, microclimate, and water availability, making it less suitable for native plants and wildlife.

- **Changes in Succession:** Invasive plants can alter the natural succession of plant communities. They may inhibit the establishment of young native plants, affecting the recovery of disturbed areas.

- **Disruption of Natural Disturbance Regimes:** Some invasive species, such as fire-adapted plants, can increase the frequency and intensity of wildfires, disrupting natural disturbance regimes and potentially harming native flora and fauna.

- **Altered Nutrient Cycling:** Invasive plants may influence nutrient cycling processes in ecosystems, affecting soil health and the availability of essential nutrients for native plants.

- **Soil Erosion:** Invasive plants can destabilize soil through changes in vegetation cover, making areas more susceptible to erosion. This can lead to sedimentation in water bodies, impacting aquatic ecosystems.

6.2 Effects on Native Wildlife

Invasive plants can have significant effects on native wildlife:

- **Altered Food Sources:** Some invasive plants provide little to no nutritional value for native herbivores, which can lead to reduced fitness and population declines in certain species.

- **Changes in Habitat Structure:** The dense growth of invasive plants can alter the physical structure of habitats, making them less suitable for native wildlife. It may impact nesting sites, shelter, and foraging opportunities.

- **Disruption of Mutualistic Relationships:** Invasive plants may not support the same pollinators, seed dispersers, and herbivores as native plants. This can disrupt mutualistic relationships between native plants and wildlife.

- **Increased Predation Risk:** Changes in habitat structure caused by invasive plants can create conditions that favor invasive predators or competitors, which can negatively affect native prey species.

- **Impacts on Rare and Endangered Species:** Invasive plants can threaten rare and endangered species by outcompeting their preferred food sources or habitat types.

6.3 Disruption of Ecosystem Services

Ecosystem services, the benefits that ecosystems provide to humans, can also be disrupted by invasive plants:

- **Water Quality:** Invasive plants can alter the hydrology of ecosystems, affecting water quality. Increased sedimentation and nutrient runoff can result from invasive species' disruption of natural vegetation.

- **Flood Control:** Changes in vegetation caused by invasive plants can impact a watershed's ability to control flooding and regulate water flow.

- **Crop and Timber Production:** Invasive plants

can invade agricultural lands and forests, reducing crop yields and timber quality. This can have economic repercussions.

- **Recreation and Aesthetics:** Invasive plants can diminish the recreational and aesthetic value of natural areas by altering their appearance and making them less enjoyable for outdoor activities.

- **Carbon Sequestration:** Some invasive plants can affect the ability of ecosystems to sequester carbon, contributing to greenhouse gas emissions and climate change.

The environmental impact of invasive plants is crucial for conservation efforts. Effective management and prevention strategies are needed to mitigate these impacts and protect native ecosystems, wildlife, and the ecosystem services upon which humans rely.

CHAPTER 7

Management and Control

7.1 Early Detection and Rapid Response

Early detection and rapid response (EDRR) are critical components of invasive plant management. Detecting and addressing invasive plants in their early stages of establishment can significantly increase the chances of successful control. Here's how EDRR works:

- **Surveillance:** Regularly monitor areas susceptible to invasive plant infestations. This includes natural areas, agricultural lands, gardens, and transportation corridors.

- **Early Identification:** Train individuals, including volunteers and professionals, to recognize invasive plants and report sightings promptly.

- **Prompt Reporting:** Encourage the public to report invasive plant sightings to local authorities or conservation organizations. Quick reporting allows for a rapid response.

- **Assessment:** Evaluate the size, extent, and severity of the infestation to determine the most appropriate control measures.

- **Prioritization:** Prioritize control efforts based on factors like the invasiveness of the species, its potential impact, and the feasibility of eradication or containment.

- **Response:** Implement control measures promptly to prevent the invasive plant from spreading further. This may involve a combination of mechanical, chemical, or biological control methods.

EDRR programs are essential for preventing the establishment and spread of invasive plants, as well as for reducing the long-term management costs associated with established infestations.

7.2 Mechanical Control Methods

Mechanical control methods involve physically removing or reducing the invasive plant population. Here are some common mechanical control techniques:

- **Manual Removal:** Hand-pulling or digging out invasive plants is effective for small infestations or isolated plants. Be sure to remove all plant parts, including roots and seeds, and dispose of them properly.

- **Mowing and Cutting:** Regular mowing or cutting can control some invasive plants. However, this method may need to be repeated multiple times, and it may stimulate resprouting.

- **Grazing:** Controlled grazing by livestock or other herbivores can help manage invasive plants, especially in grasslands and open areas. However, careful management is necessary to avoid overgrazing.

- **Prescribed Burns:** In some cases, controlled burns can be used to manage invasive plants, especially those adapted to fire-prone ecosystems. Burns should be conducted by trained professionals to ensure safety.

- **Mechanical Equipment:** Heavy machinery, such as tractors or excavators, can be used to clear large infestations. This method is often employed for invasive plants in wetlands or riparian areas.

Mechanical control methods are effective but require ongoing effort and monitoring, as invasive plants may regrow or reestablish from seeds or root fragments.

7.3 Chemical Control Methods

Chemical control methods involve the use of herbicides to kill or suppress invasive plants. Here are key considerations for chemical control:

- **Selective vs. Non-selective Herbicides:** Selective herbicides target specific plant species, while non-selective herbicides can harm a wide range of plants. Selective herbicides are preferred when native species coexist with invasive plants.

- **Application Timing:** Herbicides are most effective when applied during the plant's growth stage when it is most vulnerable. Timing depends on the species and the herbicide used.

- **Application Methods:** Herbicides can be applied as sprays, injections, or soil treatments. The choice of method depends on the target species and the surrounding environment.

- **Safety and Environmental Concerns:** Herbicide use should be carefully managed to minimize potential risks to non-target species, water sources, and human health. Follow label instructions and regulations.

- **Licensed Applicators:** In many regions, herbicides can only be applied by licensed professionals who have received training in their safe and effective use.

- **Monitoring and Follow-up:** After herbicide application, monitor the treated area to ensure the effectiveness of the control measures and to address any regrowth.

Chemical control methods can be powerful tools for managing invasive plants but should be used judiciously and in conjunction with other control measures to achieve long-term success while minimizing environmental impacts.

7.4 Biological Control

Biological control is a sustainable and environmentally friendly approach to managing invasive plants by introducing or enhancing the activity of natural enemies, such as insects, pathogens, or herbivores, that specifically target the invasive species. Here are key aspects of biological control:

- **Natural Enemies:** Biological control agents are often native insects, herbivores, or pathogens that have evolved to feed on or infect the invasive plant in its native habitat.

- **Host Specificity:** Effective biological control agents are highly host-specific, meaning they primarily target the invasive plant species and do not harm native or beneficial plants.

- **Release and Establishment:** After extensive testing and risk assessment, biological control agents are released in the invasive plant's new habitat, where they establish populations and begin to reduce the target plant's vigor and reproduction.

- **Long-Term Management:** Biological control is often considered a long-term management strategy. It may take several years for the control agent populations to build and for noticeable reductions in the invasive plant's density to occur.

- **Integrated Approach:** Biological control is most effective when integrated with other management methods, such as mechanical or chemical control, to achieve the best results.

- **Monitoring:** Ongoing monitoring is essential to assess the success of biological control and make adjustments as needed.

- **Safety and Regulation:** The release of biological control agents is regulated by government agencies to ensure that they do not pose risks to non-target species or ecosystems.

Biological control can be an effective and sustainable option for managing invasive plants, especially when the target species has become widely established and other control methods are challenging to implement. It provides a natural balance that helps restore native ecosystems by reducing the dominance of invasive plants over time. However, it is not suitable for all situations and requires careful planning and monitoring to ensure its effectiveness and safety.

CHAPTER 8

Reporting and Monitoring

8.1 How to Report Invasive Plant Sightings

Reporting invasive plant sightings is crucial for early detection and rapid response efforts to manage and control these invasive species. Here's how you can report invasive plant sightings effectively:

1. **Document the Plant:** Take clear photographs of the invasive plant, including close-up shots of leaves, flowers, and any distinguishing features.

Photographs help experts with identification.

2. **Note the Location:** Record the precise location where you observed the invasive plant. Use GPS coordinates if possible or provide detailed information about the site, such as landmarks, nearby roads, or trails.

3. **Date and Time:** Note the date and time of your observation. This information helps determine the plant's growth stage and behavior.

4. **Contact Local Authorities:** Reach out to local government agencies, conservation organizations, or invasive species management groups in your area. They often have

established protocols for reporting invasive plant sightings.

5. **Online Reporting Tools:** Many regions have online platforms or apps where you can submit invasive plant sightings. These platforms often provide guidance on what information to include.

6. **Community Science Programs:** Participate in community science programs that focus on invasive species monitoring. These programs often provide training and resources for reporting.

7. **Use Social Media:** Share your observations on social media platforms related to conservation and invasive

species. Tag relevant organizations or use appropriate hashtags to increase visibility.

8. **Educate Others:** Encourage friends, family, and neighbors to report invasive plant sightings as well. The more people who are aware of the issue, the better the chances of early detection and management.

Remember that prompt reporting is essential for effective management and prevention of invasive plants. Even if you are unsure about the identification, it is still valuable to report any suspicious plants so that experts can investigate further.

8.2 Monitoring Your Local Environment

Monitoring your local environment for invasive plants is an essential step in preventing their spread and mitigating their impacts. Here's how you can actively monitor your area:

1. **Learn to Identify Invasive Plants:** Educate yourself about common invasive plant species in your region. Familiarize yourself with their distinguishing features.

2. **Regular Walks and Hikes:** If you spend time in natural areas, take regular walks or hikes and keep an eye out for any unfamiliar plants or signs of invasive species.

3. **Join Monitoring Programs:** Participate in community-based monitoring programs focused on invasive species. These programs often provide training, guidance, and opportunities to contribute data.

4. **Document and Report:** When you encounter invasive plants, document your findings with photographs and detailed notes about the location and date. Report your observations using the methods mentioned in section 8.1.

5. **Stay Informed:** Keep up to date with local news and announcements regarding invasive species management initiatives. Attend workshops or seminars to learn more about monitoring techniques.

6. **Collaborate:** Collaborate with local conservation organizations, land managers, and government agencies involved in invasive species management. They can provide guidance and support for your monitoring efforts.

7. **Involve the Community:** Encourage your community to get involved in monitoring efforts. Organize volunteer events or awareness campaigns to raise local interest in invasive species management.

8. **Regular Follow-Up:** Conduct regular follow-up visits to the areas where you've spotted invasive plants to monitor their growth and spread. Record any changes over time.

Monitoring your local environment not only helps with early detection but also raises awareness about the importance of invasive species management in your community. By actively participating in monitoring efforts, you can contribute to the protection of native ecosystems and biodiversity.

CHAPTER 9

Prevention and Conservation

9.1 Landscape Planning to Prevent Invasions

Landscape planning plays a crucial role in preventing the spread of invasive plants and conserving native ecosystems. Here are strategies for landscape planning to prevent invasions:

1. **Choose Native Plants:**
   Prioritize native plant species in your landscaping projects. Native plants are adapted to local conditions and support native wildlife.

2. **Research Plant Selection:**
   Before adding new plants to
   your landscape, research their
   invasive potential in your
   region. Many invasive species
   are still sold in nurseries, so it's
   essential to make informed
   choices.

3. **Avoid Known Invaders:** Do
   not plant species known to be
   invasive in your area. Local
   invasive plant lists and
   guidelines can help you make
   responsible choices.

4. **Monitor Your Landscape:**
   Regularly inspect your
   landscape for any signs of
   invasive plants. Promptly
   remove and properly dispose of
   any invasive species you find.

5. **Control Escapees:** Some garden plants can become invasive if they escape cultivation. Prevent this by planting non-invasive cultivars or using physical barriers like root barriers.

6. **Reduce Disturbance:** Minimize soil disturbance during landscaping and gardening projects, as this can create opportunities for invasive plants to establish.

7. **Practice Good Hygiene:** Clean gardening tools, equipment, and footwear to prevent the unintentional spread of invasive plant seeds.

8. **Educate Others:** Share your knowledge about responsible landscaping practices with

friends, family, and neighbors to create a culture of invasive species awareness in your community.

9.2 Native Plant Gardening

Native plant gardening involves cultivating and promoting native plant species in your garden. Here's how it can contribute to invasive species prevention and conservation:

1. **Support Local Biodiversity:** Native plants attract native insects, birds, and other wildlife, contributing to local biodiversity conservation.

2. **Reduce Invasive Pressure:** By planting natives, you create healthy, biodiverse habitats that

are less susceptible to invasive species colonization.

3. **Low Maintenance:** Native plants are often well-suited to local conditions and require less water and maintenance than non-native species.

4. **Enhance Aesthetics:** Native gardens can be visually appealing and offer a sense of place, showcasing the beauty of local flora.

5. **Educational Opportunities:** Native plant gardens can serve as educational tools, helping others learn about the importance of native species and the threats posed by invasive plants.

6. **Habitat Restoration:** Consider incorporating native plants into

habitat restoration projects, such as planting native trees and shrubs in degraded areas.

9.3 Supporting Conservation Efforts

Conservation organizations and initiatives are actively working to prevent invasions and protect native ecosystems. Here's how you can support these efforts:

1. **Volunteer:** Contribute your time and energy to invasive species removal and restoration projects organized by local conservation groups.

2. **Donate:** Financially support organizations dedicated to invasive species management and conservation efforts.

3. **Advocate:** Advocate for stronger invasive species regulations and policies at the local, state, and national levels. Encourage responsible landscaping practices and invasive species prevention measures in your community.

4. **Participate in Citizen Science:** Get involved in citizen science programs focused on monitoring invasive species and collecting data for research and management.

5. **Spread Awareness:** Educate others about the importance of invasive species prevention and conservation. Host workshops, webinars, or informational sessions in your community.

6. **Collaborate:** Collaborate with local landowners, government agencies, and conservation organizations to create comprehensive invasive species management plans and conservation strategies.

Supporting conservation efforts is vital in the battle against invasive species. By working together with experts and organizations, you can contribute to the preservation of native ecosystems and the protection of biodiversity in your region.

CHAPTER 10

The Role of Beginners in Combating Invasive Plants

Beginners play a vital role in combating invasive plants, and their contributions are significant in the overall effort to manage and prevent invasive species. Here's how beginners can make a meaningful impact:

1. **Education and Awareness:** Beginners can educate themselves about common invasive plants in their region and raise awareness about the

issue among their peers, family, and community. Sharing knowledge about invasive species is the first step in prevention.

2. **Early Detection:** Beginners can actively participate in early detection efforts by keeping an eye out for invasive plants during hikes, nature walks, or while working in their gardens. Reporting sightings to local authorities or conservation organizations is critical for rapid response.

3. **Responsible Landscaping:** Beginners can make informed choices when it comes to landscaping their properties. Avoiding the use of invasive plants in gardens and landscaping projects and

replacing them with native or non-invasive alternatives is an impactful step.

4. **Supporting Conservation Organizations:** Beginners can support local conservation organizations and initiatives focused on invasive species management. These organizations often rely on volunteers and community support to carry out their work effectively.

5. **Participating in Community Efforts:** Many communities organize invasive species removal and habitat restoration events. Beginners can actively participate in these efforts, contributing their time and effort to on-the-ground actions.

6. **Advocacy:** Beginners can advocate for stronger invasive species regulations and policies in their communities. They can also encourage responsible landscaping practices and invasive species prevention measures among their neighbors and local authorities.

7. **Learning from Experts:** Beginners can seek guidance and training from experts in invasive species management. They can attend workshops, webinars, and educational events to build their knowledge and skills.

8. **Community Engagement:** Beginners can engage with their community to create a culture of invasive species awareness. This can include

organizing educational programs, workshops, and community-based invasive species monitoring initiatives.

9. **Reporting and Data Collection:** Beginners can actively participate in citizen science programs that focus on monitoring invasive species. Collecting and reporting data on invasive plant sightings can provide valuable information for management efforts.

10. **Long-Term Commitment:** Beginners can make a long-term commitment to invasive species management. Invasive plants require ongoing attention, and sustained efforts are essential for successful control and prevention.

Beginners may not have extensive experience in invasive species management, but their enthusiasm, dedication, and willingness to learn can make a significant difference in the collective effort to combat invasive plants. By taking proactive steps and collaborating with experts and experienced individuals, beginners can contribute to the preservation of native ecosystems and the protection of biodiversity.